My Hope & Focus Cancer Organizer

Manage Your Health and Ease Your Mind

by
Puja A. J. Thomson

2022 Second Revised Edition

Based on
**After Shock: From Cancer Diagnosis
to Healing**
A step-by-step guide to help you navigate your way

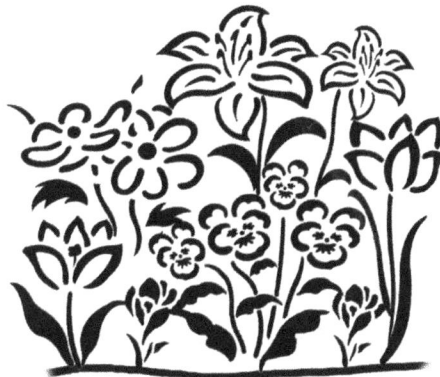

If found, please contact me and/or return to:

Name_____ Tel_____

Email: _____ Address:_____

1. Cancer   2. Health   3. Self-help

Second Revised Edition 2022   ISBN 978-1-928663-15-7

Published by—ROOTS & WINGS, New Paltz, NY. Printed in the USA

Edited by—Johanna Bard

Design—Tory Ettlinger

Logo design—Helene Sarkis

Please note: This organizer is designed with the understanding that the author and publisher are not engaged in rendering individualized professional services. The suggestions, explorations and questions are intended for individual use and are not designed to be a substitute for professional consultation.

Other works by Puja A. J. Thomson:

Track Your Truth—Discover Your Authentic Self

*My Health & Wellness Organizer—
An Easy Guide To Manage Your Healthcare—And Your Medical Records   (Revised 2022)*

After Shock: From Cancer Diagnosis to Healing (Second revisied edition 2021)

Roots & Wings for Strength and Freedom—Guided Imagery And Meditations To Transform Your Life (CD and MP3)

*Roots & Wings Workbook—Guided Imagery And Meditations To Transform Your Life
Roots & Wings (Workbook & CD)*

To order any of the above titles or for general inquiries:

845-255-2278

ROOTS & WINGS PUBLISHING, P. O. Box 1081, New Paltz, NY 12561 Email: info@rootsnwings.com

www.rootsnwings.com/store

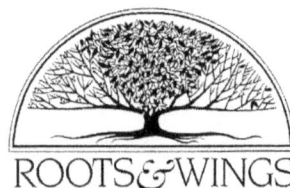

ROOTS&WINGS

CONTENTS

Foreword

My path toward becoming a breast cancer surgeon was defined in 1977 when my sister Fern was diagnosed with stage 4 breast cancer at age 35. At the time I was a junior surgical resident and I immediately shifted my attention to learning about and navigating through all Fern's treatment options, while helping to support her and our family through this tragedy. It was a powerful and overwhelming experience.

Since then I have had the honor of treating and counseling thousands of breast cancer patients. This is a tremendous responsibility and privilege. I have done my best to support their decisions while providing medically correct information in a compassionate fashion. Achieving shared medical decision-making is our goal. Providing resources that help patients organize a large amount of information as they process through their emotions and spiritual beliefs is extraordinarily important. Coordination of all treatment modalities results in optimal outcomes.

Puja Thomson's first comprehensive book *After Shock: From Cancer Diagnosis to Healing* set the ball rolling by providing an excellent road map and compass to navigate this journey. Since its publication, I have been happy to make it available to my patients who wish to participate actively in their healing process. They have found this book to be encouraging and empowering. Providing a practical framework for evaluating the pros and cons of different treatments is extremely helpful—many patients are uncertain about how to blend the best of traditional and complementary

Providing resources that help patients organize a large amount of information as they process through their emotions and spiritual beliefs is extraordinarily important.

medicine for their particular needs and beliefs. Puja's work has been a very successful tool to assist in this process.

Now Puja Thomson has created *My Hope & Focus Cancer Organizer* to enable you to keep track of everything you need to know and do during a time that may be particularly confusing or overwhelming. The organizer is a wonderful tool to simplify, sort, and arrange your decisions on treatments, health, and well-being. Confronting the large amounts of paperwork that goes with the territory can be extremely stressful. By using this organizer you will gain clarity, feel relief, reduce stress, and be able to use your energy to focus productively on your healing.

When your treatment is over, "My Survivorship Wellness Plan" offers excellent guidelines to help you and your doctor co-create a plan to assure your optimum future health and wellbeing.

Puja knows what you face from the inside out and from the outside in! I am grateful that she has drawn from her personal experience as a cancer patient and as a health care professional to develop this companion organizer. When using *My Hope & Focus Cancer Organizer*, I'm sure you will be too! Its structure will increase your confidence in your ability to play a more active role in your healing.

Sheldon Marc Feldman MD FACS
Chief, Breast Surgery and Breast Surgical Oncology and Director, Breast Cancer Services at Montefiore Medical Center; Professor of Surgery at Albert Einstein College of Medicine.

Acknowledgements

When I was wondering what to name the organizer, inspiration came from Gaitano Antonacci who had told his daughter-in-law that, for two years during his battle with melanoma, *After Shock: From Cancer Diagnosis to Healing* had given him 'hope and focus.' What better qualities and name could I wish for this organizer? Thank you, **Gaitano Antonacci,** for sharing that timely gift with me through Marisue Traina.

Many thanks go to my good friend and colleague, **Barbara Sarah LCSW,** for her unfailing encouragement. For years Barbara has been a powerhouse of inspiration in the Mid-Hudson Valley and beyond, especially as Founder of the Oncology Support Program at HealthAlliance of the Hudson Valley in Kingston NY, which continues to nurture and educate cancer patients. Through her commitment and her superb ability to network, Barbara carefully involves others in shared efforts to nurture tiny seeds into healthy flowering plants. Because of Barbara, there are so many projects and events that have seen the light of day, like this one and more recently "Circle of Friends for the Dying."

I got to know **Johanna Bard** through the Integrated Medicine Network. When she heard I was already working on an organizer based on *After Shock...,* without hesitation, she saw its purpose and offered to contribute her editing and organizational skills. Johanna's help lightened my load and our reciprocal exchange enabled me to keep my focus, sparked new insights, and led to many enjoyable moments. Thank you, Johanna.

Tory Ettlinger is much more than the skilled graphic designer of this book. Based on her personal knowledge of the challenges found in the journey from illness back to health, she has a unique sensitivity to what a user of the organizer may be experiencing. It shines through the pages. I am thankful that her design combines both clear intention and a supportive softness that has transformed the raw text in a beautiful way.

Over the past few years, it has been heart-warming and quite humbling for me to be privileged to hear the stories of many, many courageous cancer patients who have shared their experience of using *After Shock: From Cancer Diagnosis to Healing.* I thank each one of you.

Finally, I lovingly honor the memory of **Kathleen Navyo Folliard RN, Miki Frank, Joyce Goodrich PhD, and Kathleen McBryde**—four courageous women who, through cancer, have passed on beyond the limits of this life. Each contributed to *After Shock...* and to the possibility of *My Hope & Focus Cancer Organizer,* although they have not lived to see its birth.

Introduction
My Hope & Focus Cancer Organizer

If there were ever a time when I needed to weave hope and focus into my life, it was after my cancer diagnosis. I began to create a structure to support my journey. From my first fledgling notes, grew *After Shock: From Cancer Diagnosis to Healing—a step-by-step guide to help you navigate your way.* This comprehensive book is especially important during the first crucial year or when facing an unwelcome recurrence.

From that experience now comes *My Hope & Focus Cancer Organizer,* which provides a tool to simplify, sort, and organize your records.

This organizer:

❧ Removes a great deal of stress—no need to try to figure out how to arrange your paper work. It is all laid out for you.

❧ Saves lots of time.

❧ Frees your energy and contributes to your sanity—so you can more easily focus on your choices and healing.

❧ Helps you gain hope and focus as you clarify and record your journey to healing, and take charge of this "runaway train" with ease.

❧ Enables you to find information when you need it and incorporate new paperwork as it accumulates.

❧ Encourages you to be an active participant with your doctor in shaping a post-treatment survivorship wellness plan that makes sense to you.

❧ Maximizes the blessings of a healthy life while minimizing the risk of any recurrence.

There are many ways to organize your paperwork.
What matters is that <u>you</u> can find everything
—without fuss or stress.

Please note: Go to *After Shock: From Cancer Diagnosis to Healing (Second Revised Edition 2021)* for clarification of conventional and complementary treatment options, how-to's, wellness strategies and support, personal stories, and abundant resources.

HOW TO ORGANIZE YOUR INFORMATION

Use this 2022 Revision of My Hope & Focus Cancer Organizer as your master copy. The author gives you, the purchaser, for your use only, permission to make copies of those pages you will use multiple times. You may then 3-hole punch these "fill-in pages" and insert them into a 3-ring binder ready to add your information when you wish to update your medical journey.

Keep it Simple in 6 Steps

1. Fill out the ready-made forms such as "My Yellow Pages" (Pages 5-18)

2. Gather any paperwork you have already accumulated.

3. Sort it out with a support person.

 * Call a friend, family member, colleague or someone you can trust and set a time for this project.

 * Clear and reserve a space on a bookshelf for books and relevant material.

 * Put bulky items, such as articles, magazines and newsletters into folders or magazine boxes, and place them on your shelf along with books.

 * Spread all the remaining papers, (records, reports, notes) out on the top of a table or on the floor to see what you have.

 * Discard any duplicate information.

 * Sort the papers into groups of similar items such as:

   • Notes from conversations with friends

   • Questions for my professional practitioners and their answers

   • Test results

   • Bills, insurance letters and miscellaneous papers

   • Ideas and resources to follow up

 * Clip the papers of each group together.

 * Identify each group by writing its name on a brightly colored slip of paper and put that on the front page of each group.

 * Sort the papers within each group by date or by service provided.

 * Print out additional fill-in pages when you need them.

4. Insert your papers into your *Organizer* binder.

 * Create main sections using the dividers.

 * Punch holes in your papers and insert them in an appropriate section with the most recent on top.

5. Be prepared for your next appointment.
See page 50 for helpful ideas and tips.

6. Divide and conquer.

 * Use additional **dividers** to organize your paperwork more precisely so that you can find specific information more easily.

 * Use additional **binders** or one that is much thicker as your papers multiply. For example, treat this as your starter binder, and consider using a separate billing or financial binder.

PART I

MY YELLOW PAGES

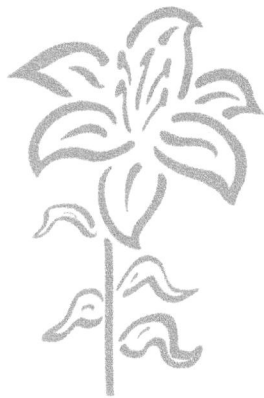

CREATING MY PERSONAL DIRECTORY

Use these pages to record all your most important cancer-related contacts to create a ready reference directory at your fingertips.

❧ **Emergency Contact and Medical Information**

❧ **Most Frequently-Used Contacts**
Make a list of the contact information you expect to refer to constantly. Knowing exactly where to turn for a particular phone number can prevent a lot of unnecessary stress.

❧ **Personal Support Team**
Individuals and Groups

❧ **Professional Team**
Doctors and Other Conventional Health Practitioners
Complementary and Alternative Medicine (CAM) Practitioners

❧ **Health Insurance, Legal and Financial Contacts**

❧ **Thank you List**—Appreciate help!

❧ **Where To Find My Important Papers / Records**—Ease your mind!

AND

❧ **Chronological Health (and Cancer) Log**
Fill out the log to the best of your ability, including your health history prior to your diagnosis, first symptoms [if any] and discovery of your cancer, through diagnosis, follow-up tests and results, treatment decisions and all appointments.)

Keep this record of your progress up-to-date. Include any other health concerns. Refer to it during an office visit. You will not have to rack your brain to remember details, and it may prevent you from blanking out, when physicians ask for such information.

Make sure you continually update these pages.

*What matters is that you know where to find everything
—at the drop of a hat!*

EMERGENCY CONTACTS AND MEDICAL INFORMATION

Add your emergency telephone contact numbers below and add your primary ICE (In Case of Emergency) numbers to your cell phone contact list.

	NAME	HOME PHONE	CELL PHONE	WORK PHONE

Primary contact:_____

If unavailable, contact:_____

Next of kin _____

Friend _____

Walk-In Medical Clinic/
Hospital Emergency Room _____

Police, Fire, Ambulance
(if in doubt, call 911) _____

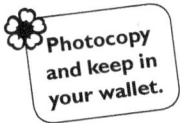

Photocopy and keep in your wallet.

EMERGENCY MEDICAL DATA

Name: _____

Phone: _____

Insurance Co. and ID#: _____

Emergency Contact: _____ Phone:_____

Doctor's Name:_____ Phone _____

Medical Conditions:_____

Medications:_____ Blood Group: _____

Medication Allergies: _____

Additional Information:

_____

_____

_____

_____

_____

_____

_____

_____

_____

MOST FREQUENTLY USED CONTACTS

Put an asterisk * next to the person who is willing to coordinate your treatment.

Name	Telephone / Cell	Email

PERSONAL SUPPORT: INDIVIDUALS AND GROUPS

Fill this in after you 1) have made your decisions using the guidelines in Part Two, and 2) have agreement from those whom you have asked. Identify any special role such as a patient navigator or spokesperson for other team members.

INDIVIDUALS (close family, friends, clergy)

Name	Best way to contact - Telephone / Cell	Email	Address

GROUPS (centers, support groups, organizations)

Name	Best way to contact - Telephone / Cell	Email	Address

PROFESSIONAL TEAM
MEDICAL DOCTORS AND OTHER CONVENTIONAL HEALTH PRACTITIONERS

Include your primary and other doctors, nurses, specialists, oncology support contacts as you enlist them.

Put an asterisk * next to the person who will coordinate your treatment.

Primary Care Physician _____ My patient #_____

Name of office _____ Insurance accepted YES / NO

Address _____

Best way to contact office: Tel _____ Fax_____ Email _____

Receptionist and / or Secretary _____ Nurse _____

Hospital affiliation _____ Has copy of living will and health care proxy YES / NO

Oncologist _____ My patient #_____

Name of office _____ Insurance accepted YES / NO

Address _____

Best way to contact office: Tel _____ Fax_____ Email _____

Receptionist and / or Secretary _____ Nurse _____

Hospital affiliation _____ Has copy of living will and health care proxy YES / NO

Surgeon _____ My patient #_____

Name of office _____ Insurance accepted YES / NO

Address _____

Best way to contact office: Tel _____ Fax _____ Email _____

Receptionist and / or Secretary _____ Nurse _____

Hospital affiliation _____ Has copy of living will and health care proxy YES / NO

Radiologist _____ My patient #_____

Name of office _____ Insurance accepted YES / NO

Address _____

Best way to contact office: Tel _____ Fax _____ Email _____

Receptionist and / or Secretary _____ Nurse _____

Hospital affiliation _____ Has copy of living will and health care proxy YES / NO

Second Opinion _____ My patient #_____

Name of office _____ Insurance accepted YES / NO

Address _____

Best way to contact office: Tel _____ Fax _____ Email _____

Receptionist and / or Secretary _____ Nurse _____

Hospital affiliation _____ Has copy of living will and health care proxy YES / NO

PROFESSIONAL TEAM
COMPLEMENTARY, ALTERNATIVE AND INTEGRATIVE MEDICAL PRACTITIONERS

Include your holistic doctors, nurses, acupuncturists, naturopaths, healers, massage therapists, chiropractors, cranial-sacral body workers, counselors and others.

Put an asterisk * next to the person who is willing to coordinate your medical care.

Name_____ My patient #_____

Modality _____

Name of office _____ Insurance accepted   YES / NO

Address_____

Best way to contact office: Tel _____ Fax _____ Email _____

Receptionist and/or Secretary_____ Nurse_____

Hospital affiliation_____ Has copy of living will and health care proxy YES / NO

Name_____ My patient #_____

Modality _____

Name of office _____ Insurance accepted YES / NO

Address_____

Best way to contact office: Tel _____ Fax _____ Email _____

Receptionist and/or Secretary_____ Nurse_____

Hospital affiliation_____ Has copy of living will and health care proxy YES / NO

Name_____ My patient #_____

Modality _____

Name of office _____ Insurance accepted YES / NO

Address_____

Best way to contact office: Tel _____ Fax _____ Email _____

Receptionist and/or Secretary_____ Nurse_____

Hospital affiliation_____ Has copy of living will and health care proxy YES / NO

Name_____ My patient #_____

Modality _____

Name of office _____ Insurance accepted YES / NO

Address_____

Best way to contact office: Tel _____ Fax _____ Email _____

Receptionist and/or Secretary_____ Nurse_____

Hospital affiliation_____ Has copy of living will and health care proxy YES / NO

PROFESSIONAL TEAM
INSURANCE, LEGAL, AND FINANCIAL CONTACTS

HEALTH INSURANCE

Primary Health Insurance Company _____

Membership ID _____ Effective date _____

Plan name _____ Policy / group number _____

Contact person, if any _____ Tel / fax / email _____

Secondary Health Insurance Company _____

Membership ID _____ Effective date _____

Plan name _____ Policy / group number _____

Contact person, if any _____ Tel / fax / email _____

Other Insurance, such as long-term care

Membership ID _____ Effective date _____

Plan name _____ Policy / group number _____

Contact person, if any _____ Tel / fax / email _____

LEGAL

Healthcare Proxy _____

Address _____

Tel / fax / email _____ Relationship _____

Has copy of my healthcare proxy form   YES / NO

Lawyer _____

Address _____

Tel / fax / email _____ Office receptionist, if any _____

Has copy of my will, living will and healthcare proxy form   YES / NO

Power of Attorney _____

Address _____

Tel / fax / email _____ Relationship _____

Has copy of my will, living will and healthcare proxy form   YES / NO

Back-up Health Care Proxy / PoA _____

Telephone / email _____

Relationship _____

PROFESSIONAL TEAM
INSURANCE, LEGAL, AND FINANCIAL CONTACTS (cont'd)

Additional People (eg Family Members, Doctors) Who Have a Copy of My Legal Papers

Name	Will	Living will	Healthcare proxy
_____	☐	☐	☐
_____	☐	☐	☐
_____	☐	☐	☐
_____	☐	☐	☐
_____	☐	☐	☐
_____	☐	☐	☐

FINANCIAL

Financial Advisor _____

Office address_____

Office receptionist, if any _____ Tel / fax / email _____

Tax Preparer/Accountant _____

Office address_____

Office receptionist, if any _____ Tel / fax / email _____

Bank _____ **Manager** _____

Address_____

Best contact info_____

Other _____

Address_____

Best contact info_____

THANK YOU LIST

Here you can keep a record of any gifts of love, or kind thoughtful actions, no matter how small, as well as when and how you have expressed your gratitude.

Person to thank + contact info	For call / card / email	Thanked by Date

WHERE TO FIND MY IMPORTANT PAPERS / RECORDS

For ease of mind, list where you keep all your important information. Once completed, provide a copy for your lawyer and close family members. LAST UPDATED:_____

Item	Located in						
	Bank safety deposit box	Home firebox	Home filing cabinet	Office	Lawyer	Wallet	Other
Computer Passwords							
Back up drive							
Financial							
Bank accounts							
Credit card info.							
IOUs							
IRAs / Roths							
Investments							
Retirement and pension							
Tax returns							
Other							
House / Home							
Deed / Mortgage							
Rental							
Other							
Insurance							
Car (+ title, registration)							
Health							
House / rental							
Other							
Legal							
Healthcare proxy							
Living will							
Organ donor info.							
Power of Attorney							
Will / Trust							
Other							
Personal							
Birth certificate							
Divorce/separation papers							
Driver's license							
Funeral arrangements							
Marriage certificate							
Passport							
Social Security Number							
Other							

CHRONOLOGICAL HEALTH HISTORY

Create an overview of your general medical information to the best of your ability. You will be able to give a copy to all your health care providers when they request it.

GENERAL MEDICAL INFORMATION

Today's date (mm /dd /yyyy)_____

Name _____ Age _____ Date of birth _____

Street _____ City _____ State _____ Zip _____

Home tel _____ Cell tel _____ Work tel_____

Blood type _____ Social Security # _____

Next of kin /emergency contact _____ Best way to reach _____

Health Care Proxy _____ Best way to reach_____

Allergies (with medications, if any) _____

Vital signs, recorded by staff before you meet a doctor:

DATE	Weight	Height	Blood Pressure	Pulse
_____	_____	_____	_____	_____
_____	_____	_____	_____	_____
_____	_____	_____	_____	_____
_____	_____	_____	_____	_____
_____	_____	_____	_____	_____

Previous surgeries, if any, with dates_____

_____

Other medical conditions and medications _____

_____

Any other information you think is important_____

PAST / CURRENT FAMILY HISTORY

List significant illness(es) and / or cause of death for immediate family members:

Mother _____

Father _____

Siblings _____

CHRONOLOGICAL HEALTH HISTORY (cont'd)

SOCIAL & HEALTH HISTORY

Occupation _____

Marital status _____

Please list the amount consumed:

Alcoholic beverages per day _____ / week _____ Cigarettes per day _____ / week _____

Glasses of soda per day _____ / week _____ How often do you exercise per week? _____ times

How many hours sleep do you generally get per night? _____ hours

Do you wear your seat belt regularly?   Yes   No

Have you experienced problems with any of the following? If yes, please explain below.

Heart / Vascular	☐ no	☐ yes*
Breathing	☐ no	☐ yes
Stomach / Intestines	☐ no	☐ yes
Female / Male Organs	☐ no	☐ yes
Kidney / Bladder	☐ no	☐ yes
Brain / Spinal Cord	☐ no	☐ yes
Muscles / Joints / Bone	☐ no	☐ yes
Thyroid	☐ no	☐ yes
Skin	☐ no	☐ yes
Cancerous Growths	☐ no	☐ yes

*Explanation of any of the above: _____

_____

_____

_____

CURRENT HEALTH CHALLENGE:

Chief complaint: _____

When did you first notice something was wrong? _____

What did you experience? _____

Circle severity of pain on scale   1   2   3   4   5   6   7   8   9   10

(1 = hardly noticeable and 10 = most severe)

Other Comments _____

CHRONOLOGICAL CANCER LOG

FIRST CANCER DIAGNOSIS_____ Date (mm/dd/yyyy) _____

Given by _____

Facility _____

Doctor's Follw-up recommendations_____

My response _____

Additional consultations, 2nd opinions and tests to help me decide my treatment

Health Professional _____ Date _____

    Facility _____

    Purpose _____

    Findings/recommendations _____

    _____ Reports / tests filed under _____

Health Professional _____ Date _____

    Facility _____

    Purpose _____

    Findings/recommendations _____

    _____ Reports / tests filed under _____

Health Professional _____ Date _____

    Facility _____

    Purpose _____

    Findings/recommendations _____

    _____ Reports / tests filed under _____

Health Professional _____ Date _____

    Facility _____

    Purpose _____

    Findings/recommendations _____

    _____ Reports / tests filed under _____

CHRONOLOGICAL CANCER LOG (cont'd)

MY CURRENT TREATMENT DECISION(S) _____ Date (mm/dd/yyyy) _____

Remember to review PART 2 before making ANY decisions!

FIRST TREATMENT Date _____ Location _____

With _____ or under the supervision of _____

Treatment / tests given _____ Reports / tests filed under_____

Medication(s) prescribed _____

Notes _____

FURTHER TREATMENTS / APPOINTMENTS

Add all consultations, tests and test results, adjuvant therapies, alternative therapies, chemotherapy drugs, and prescribed medications in chronological order under the headings below:

Date _____ Reason for visit _____

With _____ or under the supervision of _____

Treatment / tests given _____ Reports / tests filed under_____

Medication(s) prescribed _____

Notes _____

Date _____ Reason for visit _____

With _____ or under the supervision of _____

Treatment / tests given _____ Reports / tests filed under_____

Medication(s) prescribed _____

Notes _____

Date _____ Reason for visit _____

With _____ or under the supervision of _____

Treatment / tests given _____ Reports / tests filed under_____

Medication(s) prescribed _____

Notes _____

CHRONOLOGICAL CANCER LOG (cont'd)

FURTHER TREATMENTS / APPOINTMENTS

Date _____ Reason for Visit_____

With _____ or under the supervision of _____

Treatment / tests given _____ Reports / tests filed under _____

Medication(s) prescribed _____

Notes _____

Date _____ Reason for Visit_____

With _____ or under the supervision of _____

Treatment / tests given _____ Reports / tests filed under _____

Medication(s) prescribed _____

Notes _____

Date _____ Reason for Visit_____

With _____ or under the supervision of _____

Treatment / tests given _____ Reports / tests filed under _____

Medication(s) prescribed _____

Notes _____

Date _____ Reason for Visit_____

With _____ or under the supervision of _____

Treatment / tests given _____ Reports / tests filed under _____

Medication(s) prescribed _____

Notes _____

Date _____ Reason for Visit_____

With _____ or under the supervision of _____

Treatment / tests given _____ Reports / tests filed under _____

Medication(s) prescribed _____

Notes _____

PART 2

DECISIONS, DECISIONS, DECISIONS

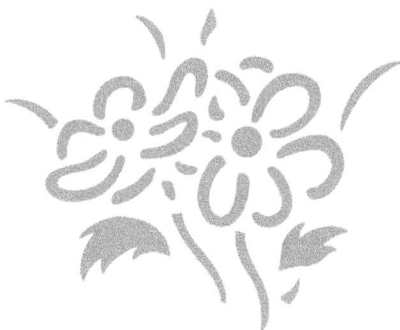

MAKE PERSONAL SUPPORT DECISIONS

You may not initially know if you need help or what your needs will be or even how to ask for help and from whom, but when you do...

USE THE QUESTIONS on the following pages to help you clarify the kind of support you wish to have.

Ask yourself how you'd like your family, friends and community to support you with specific tasks. (These may be different from what people offer you). It's important to identify the help you *do* need and make your decisions. You can gently refuse help you do not need. List those whom you wish to ask.

TAKE ACTION

❀ Invite those you have chosen to help you.

❀ Ask for what you need; this is not a time to go it alone.

❀ Delegate.

❀ Add the contact information of those who have agreed to be on your "*Personal Support Team*" on page 7 in *My Yellow Pages*. (Remember that too many people can be overwhelming, and it can be helpful to choose a spokesperson).

UPDATE FROM TIME TO TIME

❀ Review your personal wellness progress (Page 26)

A FEW PRETTY GOOD TIPS

WHEN MAKING DECISIONS

Following the shock of your diagnosis, you may be in turmoil and not know how best to make decisions.

* VERY IMPORTANT!
This is a perfect time to reach out to the trusted people in your life, be they family, friends, professionals or a cancer survivor / patient navigator to help you navigate these challenging issues and daunting questions. This is not a time to go it alone.

❀ It is important to clarify your preferences by noting both your thoughts and feelings *before* you make any decisions.

❀ *Please take your time.*

❀ Give yourself a break between each question.

❀ Ask your helper to go through it with you, and if it is easier for you, ask him or her to make a note of your answers.

If this feels overwhelming to you, just do what you can.

WHAT ARE MY NEEDS AT THIS TIME?

What practical support would I most appreciate?
E.g. Errands, child care, special food, driving to appointments?

What emotional support would I most appreciate?
E.g. Call after appointments, listen, help me look at options?

What spiritual support would I most appreciate?
E.g. Set up prayer circle, inspirational readings, walk with friend, connect with spiritual mentor?

What would **NOT** be of help to me?
E.g. Constant invasive phone questions, lasagna (if that's not a food I like)?

How can I best ask for what I do need?
E.g. Be honest with self, and then with others?

HOW CAN FAMILY AND FRIENDS HELP ME MEET THESE NEEDS?

What are the strengths of my close family members and friends?

Who   What

_____

_____

_____

_____

Who is good at doing what?

Who   What

_____

_____

_____

_____

What have my family members and friends offered to do, if anything?

Who   What

_____

_____

_____

_____

How would I like them to be involved?

Who   What

_____

_____

_____

_____

Would I benefit from having someone in a special role such as spokesperson, to pass on information to other team members? If so, how?

WHAT OTHER COMMUNITY SUPPORT WOULD BE HELPFUL TO ME?

Support / patient group

Religious / spiritual organization

Internet

Blog

Social network

Chat group

Other...

HOW WOULD I LIKE OTHERS TO HELP ME?

Prioritize and list your needs.

Make a couple of copies: one to put on the fridge or beside your phone and one to carry with you, so you won't draw a blank when you are asked what help you need.

Help I need	When? now or later / date	Person I'll ask / who offered	Ongoing or done?

MY PERSONAL SUPPORT TEAM

List those special people you wish to invite to be members of your personal support team.

Add their contact information to *My Personal Support Team* page in *My Yellow Pages*, when they have agreed.
*Remember to identify your spokesperson, if you have one.

Name	Phone #	Date invited	To help with	Now/later

REVIEW MY PERSONAL WELLNESS PROGRESS FROM TIME TO TIME

A good time to review your personal wellness progress is when you review your medical healthcare progress.

Can I say "yes" to the following statements?

1. I am eliminating as much stress as possible.

2. I have confidence in my doctors and in my treatment.

3. I am keeping the scheduled appointments and treatments that I have committed to.

4. I will persevere even when things are difficult.

5. I believe I will be among those who survive my kind of cancer.

6. I am now ready to make changes in my lifestyle to increase my chances of wellness, for example:

Check those that you can commit to at this time:

☐ relaxation

☐ meditation

☐ guided imagery

☐ singing

☐ painting or being creative by
_____

☐ listening to music

☐ appreciation of beauty

☐ connecting to nature

☐ walking

☐ exercise by _____

☐ wholesome diet, limiting / giving up alcohol, tobacco, sugar

☐ people I love to be with_____
_____

☐ things I love to do _____

☐ resurrecting an old hobby

☐ massage and / or body work

☐ having naps

☐ pampering myself by _____
_____

☐ writing in my journal*

☐ dreams—short-term and / or long-term goals
_____

☐ laughter

☐ gratitude

☐ movies

☐ gardening

☐ time alone

☐ other ways to love and appreciate my life
_____

Make a schedule with notes about how and when you will follow through on these choices.

*This could also be a good time to re-read personal notes if you keep a journal. Some people find doing so really helpful.

Keep going step-by-step and congratulate yourself!

Remember to reach out to someone for encouragement and support when you need it.

MAKE TREATMENT DECISIONS AND ENLIST PROFESSIONAL SUPPORT

Decide initial treatment preferences
Refine treatment choices
Sharpen *focus* towards a more considered opinion
Finalize treatment decisions
Choose professional team

If you have already agreed to a treatment plan, or your feel this section does not apply to you, please SKIP it for now and move the pages of this section to the back of your book.

TAKE ACTION

Identify and invite the professionals whom you wish to be responsible for the treatments you have chosen.

Add the contact information for each to your Yellow Pages, when they have agreed.

Ask yourself, **"Who will coordinate my treatment?"**

This person will oversee your total treatment plan. Your primary physician is often the most appropriate choice for conventional cancer care. Choose someone you are comfortable with. If that person is not able to do so, ask for another referral.

The person who has agreed to coordinate my treatment is

Name: Best way to contact:

If you can't find such a willing person, use *My Hope & Focus Cancer Organizer*, with your notes and your questions, as a resource to help you be your own overseer—and your own advocate.

Take your binder to appointments as a reminder that cancer care can be a coordinated service.

TAKE YOUR TIME

It is important to clarify your preferences by noting both your thoughts and feelings before you make any treatment decisions or enlist the support of any practitioner. However, please take your time. Hasty decisions may not be in your best interests. If this thorough approach feels overwhelming to you, just do what you can.

⊛ Give yourself a break between the steps that follow.

⊛ Ask a friend or family member to go through it with you, and perhaps make a note of your answers.

⊛ Do whatever feels useful to you in order to be ready to select your treatment and professional team…and leave the rest.

WHAT DO I PREFER?
DECIDE INITIAL TREATMENT PREFERENCES

1. What kinds of diagnostic tools and interventions have worked for me in the past?

2. For my specific cancer diagnosis, what do I see to be the benefits and strengths of:
- Conventional medicine?

- Complementary and alternative care?

- A combination of conventional and complementary modalities- Integrative medicine?

3. How confident, comfortable, and hopeful do I feel treating my cancer with recommendations and prescriptions of:
- Conventional physicians?

- Complementary and alternative care practitioners?

- Integrative practitioners (a combination of conventional and complementary modalities)?

REFINE TREATMENT CHOICES

Use the following charts to further clarify your initial treatment preferences by checking the appropriate box below.

Conventional Options

TESTS

	YES I'm comfortable using this test	**NO** I'm not interested	**DON'T KNOW** Want more info
Biopsy	☐	☐	☐
Blood sample analysis	☐	☐	☐
Cat Scan or CT Scan	☐	☐	☐
Genetic Testing	☐	☐	☐
Mammography	☐	☐	☐
MRI	☐	☐	☐
Palpating	☐	☐	☐
PETscan	☐	☐	☐
Radiographic studies (X-ray)	☐	☐	☐
Ultrasound	☐	☐	☐
Other_____	☐	☐	☐

TREATMENTS

	YES I'm comfortable using this treatment	**NO** I'm not interested	**DON'T KNOW** Want more info
Biopsy	☐	☐	☐
Chemotherapy	☐	☐	☐
Drugs	☐	☐	☐
Immunotherapy	☐	☐	☐
Irradiation	☐	☐	☐
Radiotherapy	☐	☐	☐
Surgery	☐	☐	☐
Other _____	☐	☐	☐

REFINE TREATMENT CHOICES (cont'd)

Complementary Options

TESTS

	YES I'm comfortable using this test	**NO** I'm not interested	**DON'T KNOW** I want more info
Biofeedback	☐	☐	☐
Detailed life history	☐	☐	☐
Eye, tongue and skin exam	☐	☐	☐
Genetic testing	☐	☐	☐
Muscle testing	☐	☐	☐
Pulses	☐	☐	☐
Thermography	☐	☐	☐
Other_____	☐	☐	☐

TREATMENTS

	YES I'm comfortable using this test	**NO** I'm not interested	**DON'T KNOW** I want more info
Acupuncture	☐	☐	☐
Aromatherapy	☐	☐	☐
Ayurvedic	☐	☐	☐
Bach flower essences	☐	☐	☐
Biofeedback	☐	☐	☐
Chiropractic	☐	☐	☐
Energy healing	☐	☐	☐
Essential oils	☐	☐	☐
Health kinesiology	☐	☐	☐
Holistic nursing	☐	☐	☐
Homeopathy	☐	☐	☐
Massage therapy	☐	☐	☐
Meditation	☐	☐	☐
Mental health counseling	☐	☐	☐
Naturopathy	☐	☐	☐
Nutritional / herbal counseling	☐	☐	☐
Osteopathic manipulation	☐	☐	☐
Physical therapy	☐	☐	☐
Reflexology	☐	☐	☐
Spiritual healing	☐	☐	☐
Tai Chi	☐	☐	☐
Traditional Chinese medicine	☐	☐	☐
Yoga	☐	☐	☐
Other _____	☐	☐	☐

SHARPEN FOCUS TOWARDS A MORE CONSIDERED OPINION

1. **Add up your Yesses. Note where most are on your chart.**

   Number of Conventional Yesses _____   Number of Complementary/Alternative Yesses_____

2. **Consider all the information you have thus far gained from your experience, discussions and research, and ask:**

   Given my type of cancer, what are my reasons for:

   - choosing conventional treatments?

   - choosing complementary and / or alternative treatments?

   - choosing to integrate conventional and complementary treatments?

3. **Ask, "What else would I like to know before making a fully informed choice?"**

   For example, do I need to ask more questions such as:

   - What is the advice of my physician and / or my Complementary and Alternative Medicine (CAM) health provider?

   - Have I been given any choices of treatment? If not, ask to initiate that discussion.

   - What conventional treatments have been specifically recommended for my condition?

   - What complementary / alternative treatments have been specifically recommended?

   - What treatments are congruent with my perspectives about healing?

   - What is the evidence in support of all these specific recommendations?

   - What do clinical trials, if any, of patients with my type and stage of cancer show about such treatments?

4. **Tap into your intuition**

   I will take time to slow down, e.g. by walking in nature, so that I can feel my inner response to each possibility, and ask, "What is my gut feeling now about each approach?"

SHARPEN FOCUS TOWARDS A MORE CONSIDERED OPINION (cont'd)

If I need further information about a specific question or concern noted on the previous page, I will call on the appropriate resource/person to help me get the pertinent information.

Issue / Question	Possible Resource	Person to ask for assistance
	Library The Internet Organizations Local support groups Other _____	
	Library The Internet Organizations Local support groups Other _____	
	Library The Internet Organizations Local support groups Other _____	
	Library The Internet Organizations Local support groups Other _____	

Research notes

FINALIZE TREATMENT DECISIONS

❧ **What is my considered judgment now about what would help my body heal…**

…from conventional medicine?

…from complementary care?

…from alternative care?

❧ **Does this feel right to me?**

❧ **I now choose the following modalities for treatment:**

Initially:

Along with:

Followed by:

CHOOSING MY PROFESSIONAL TEAM

HEALTH PROFESSIONALS WHO ARE ALREADY ON MY TEAM:

Name of Physician or Health Professional	Area of Expertise

ADDITIONAL PROFESSIONAL SUPPORT I NEED

Ask yourself, "What other specialists or professional skills do I need for my healing"?

List those you need below (e.g. an oncologist? an acupuncturist?)

Ask for recommendations and leads.

Area of Expertise	Physician or Health Professional Suggested	Recommended By

FOR EACH SPECIALIST, ASK WHAT CRITERIA IS MOST IMPORTANT TO ME?

	Very important	Important	Not a concern
Training and qualifications*			
Professional reputation and peer reviews			
Distance—how far am I willing to travel?			
Openness to communicate with other professionals			
Ability to listen to my questions and communicate clearly			
Staff and facility welcoming and approachable			
Other (For example, will my insurance be accepted?)			

*Make sure any physician is "Board Certified" in their specialty

CHOOSING MY PROFESSIONAL TEAM (Cont'd)

Record the results of your inquiries. Then note your decision whether to continue with each practitioner.

Name	Specialty	Date contacted	By phone or in person	Decided to follow up: YES / NO

❧ **If you feel hopeful, supported and compatible with a practitioner you've contacted, and you are ready to follow up with this practitioner, invite them to become a member of your professional team. Then add his or her contact information to your Professional List in *My Yellow Pages*.**

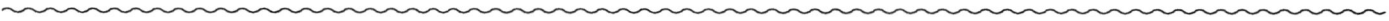

PART 3

MY MEDICAL APPOINTMENTS

MAKING THE MOST OF MY MEDICAL APPOINTMENTS
Prepare detailed questions in advance

BEFORE ANY MEDICAL APPOINTMENT (for a diagnosis, consultation or test result):

Ask yourself, "What do I want to know about my diagnosis and my treatment options?"

> *Highlight* the questions listed on the following pages that you wish to ask about your diagnosis or about a specific treatment.
>
> *Cross out* those you do not wish to ask.
>
> *Add* any others.
>
> *Adapt* these questions for your type of cancer and for possible treatments, such as radiation.

PREPARING MY QUESTIONS

Prepare thoroughly in advance to get the most out of your medical visits:

- ❀ **Plan ahead to invite a member of your personal support team or a local advocacy group to go with you, if post-Covid mandates allow this. Otherwise ask permission to record specific info.**

- ❀ Review, reorder and regroup **your questions / concerns.**

- ❀ Go through the list systematically to make sure that you have nothing left to check or if the wording could be more precise. It's your right to have your questions answered, but physicians are very busy people. Be as succinct and clear as possible. If your questions are clear, your doctors' answers can be more focused and helpful.

- ❀ Make extra copies of the list to take with you, one for the person accompanying you and one for your physician or health professional, if you wish him or her to have it.

- ❀ **Respect the limits of what you can comfortably handle at any one time as you do this preparation.** Take breaks and enlist help **so that you don't get overwhelmed.** While it is normal to feel overwhelmed, being well prepared will build your confidence.

AT YOUR IN-PERSON OR TELEMEDICINE (TELEONCOLOGY) VISIT

Ask the doctor your questions, and ask your companion / navigator to note the answers.

QUESTIONS about...

MY DIAGNOSIS

Dr._____Date (mmddyyyy) _____

Q: What exactly is my diagnosis?
A:

Q: Would you please describe my condition in simple language?
A:

Q: How did you arrive at your opinion? How certain are you?
A:

Q: What symptoms have you observed or have I reported to you that led to your diagnosis?
A:

Q: Could there be other reasons for my symptoms?
A:

Q: How will this diagnosis affect my life?
A:

Q: Will I have to make any changes day to day?
A:

Q: What must I now take into consideration? Do I need to be alert for symptoms in any other part of my body?
A:

Q: What are your specific recommendations regarding next steps?
A:

MY TESTS AND RESULTS

Dr. _____ Date (mmddyyyy) _____

Q: What tests support your diagnosis? What specific information did this test (_____) show?
A:

Q: What is the size of the malignant area in centimeters? ((1 cm))
A:

Q: What is the grade of cells (aggressiveness of cells)? What does that mean?
A:

Q: Are the malignant cells fast moving or slow moving? Hard to destroy, or easy to destroy? Hard to remove or easy to remove? What does that mean?
A:

Q: Do you already know the answers to these questions from the lab test or pathology report? If not, then when will you know?
A:

Q: Are there any supportive tests that can tell me more about my tumor, e.g. estrogen receptor status?
A:

Q: Has the cancer spread to any other place(s) in my body? If so, where?
A:

Q: What other sites have been checked for cancer and found cancer-free?
A:

Q: Do I need further tests? If so, is the test you are recommending necessary to identify the type of cancer I have?
A:

Q: Will this test that you are recommending help you (the doctor) or me, come to a more informed decision? What will the test entail?
A:

☙ **Question for myself** (and discuss with a support person):
Q: Are the health professionals I've consulted in agreement with each other?
A:

MY TREATMENT OPTIONS

Dr. _____ Date (mmddyyyy) _____

Q: What are my treatment options?
A:

Q: Which of these are standard treatments? And with which have you had success?
A:

Q: Are there alternatives? If so, what?
A:

Q: For each possible option, please tell me where the treatment will be given.
What is the duration of the treatment? How often will it be given?
A:

Q: What are the **benefits** of this treatment?	Short-term?	Long-term?
A:		

Q: What are the **risks** of this treatment?	Short-term?	Long-term?
A:		

Q: What are the **side effects** of this treatment?	Short-term?	Long-term?
A:		

Q: Do you know of any experimental treatments or clinical trials for my kind of cancer that you would
recommend for me?
A:

Q: Is it better to get a second opinion now before anything is done, or wait till after the tests, surgery
or other procedures that you may be recommending? Why?
A:

✿ **Question for myself** (and discuss with a support person):
Q: Do I have enough information? If not, what is lacking?
A:

QUESTIONS
about...

MY DOCTOR'S RECOMMENDATIONS

Dr. _____ Date (mmddyyyy) _____

Q: What are your specific recommendations?
A:

Q: What are your reasons for recommending _____?
A:

Q: How did you decide which treatment(s) to recommend to me?
A:

Q: What flexibility do I have?
A:

Q: Can you point to research that would give me confidence in the specific intervention(s) you are recommending for my kind of cancer?
A:

Q: Where might I learn more about this method of treating my particular cancer?
A:

Q: Is there anything else I need to know?
A:

QUESTIONS
about...

TIMING OF RECOMMENDED TREATMENTS

Dr. _____ Date (mmddyyyy) _____

Q: What decisions regarding treatment do you recommend I must make NOW—before I leave your office or within 24-48 hours? Why?
A:

Q: How life-threatening is my diagnosis?
A:

Q: What decisions must I make SOON?
A:

Q: How soon?
A:

Q: What decisions can I make LATER?
A:

Q: How long may I wait before I have to decide?
A:

Q: If you are recommending a later decision, why is that?
A:

Q: Does a specific treatment have to come after or before another treatment?
A:

Q: What amount of "wiggle-room" do I have to do further research, without being pressured by fear or time constraints?
A:

Q: How long is the treatment? And how lengthy is the recuperation?
A:

Questions for myself (and discuss with a support person)

Q: If a physician is recommending immediate treatment within a few days, do I understand, and agree with, this urgency as a medical necessity?
A:

Q: Have I had enough time to absorb the shock and make peace with my decision?
A:

Q: Do I need more information before deciding? If so, what and from whom?
A:

QUESTIONS
about...

MY OTHER CONCERNS

Dr. _____ Date (mmddyyyy) _____

Q: Given your experience, what is the general life expectancy with this type of cancer at this stage? Be truthful, please. (I understand that no one can predict exactly what any outcome will be, and nor can statistics.)

A:

Q: What is your definition of remission? How will I know if I am in remission? Is it disease-free for, say, 5 years?

A:

Q: What is your definition of cure? How will I know if I am cured? For how long can I expect to be disease-free?—say, 3–5 years, or for the rest of my life, or what?

A:

Q: Is my cancer linked to any other kind of cancer? Is increased vigilance needed in any other part of my body?

A:

Q: Do you recommend any complementary treatments to integrate with your protocol?

A:

Q: Do you have any suggestions as to how I can support my healing? For example with diet, acupuncture, massage, support groups, nutrition or other complementary modalities for my type of cancer? If so, can you recommend any research on any of the above?

A

Q: I know you can't see into the future, but from your medical training what is the likely course of events if I do nothing?

A:

Q: Does the hospital have a tissue bank? How long do they save the tissue and slides after a biopsy or surgery?

A:

Q: If I need treatment in a medical facility, where will it be—in your office or in a hospital?

A:

Other Questions _____

A:

QUESTIONS for...

MY SURGEON (Example—Breast Cancer Surgeon)

Dr. _____ Date (mmddyyyy) _____

Q: What is a "lumpectomy"? Is it only the "cancer" cells that will be removed?

A:

Q: How large an area around the cancer will be cut out to ensure that all the cancer tissue is removed? (What will the margins be?)

A:

Q: Will you take out any lymph nodes? If so, under what circumstances would you remove them? What about sentinel nodes?

A:

Q: What is the statistical recurrence of cancer after a lumpectomy?

A:

Q: How will my mobility be affected? How soon after surgery can I take part in sports and other indoor or outdoor physical activities?

A:

Q: At what point do you recommend a lumpectomy? Is it possible for my body to handle this itself since my body is a self-repairing system? In my case, is it possible to delay a lumpectomy, if I take measures to support my body's capacity to work on bringing about healing? And how can I best support that? Can you suggest any other treatments now available as a result of new research such as the Human Genome Project? Immunotherapy?

A:

Q: You've mentioned following up with radiation / chemotherapy / _____. Why is it a necessary part of the treatment? What would this achieve?

A:

Q: What are the chances of this treatment damaging my heart or my _____? What are the other possible side effects?

A:

Q: What do statistics show when comparing results with or without radiation? After five years? After ten years or longer? Likewise for Tamoxifen and chemotherapy.

A:

QUESTIONS
for...

MY MEDICAL ONCOLOGIST

Dr. _____ Date (mmddyyyy) _____

BEFORE CHEMOTHERAPY

Q: Am I among those who would benefit from chemotherapy, or not, according to genomic testing?
YES / NO

Q: What chemotherapy drugs will be used?

A: Name of drug	Benefits	Potential side effects

Q: How many treatments will I receive? And how might I expect to feel after each treatment?
A:

Q: Will I need a port, shunt or catheter to receive the treatment? Please explain. Should I expect to experience any pain or discomfort?
A:

Q: Who will monitor my progress? How? And whom may I consult if I experience any problems with side effects?
A:

Q: What will the long-term effects be?
A:

Q: How will I know if the treatments are working?
A:

Q: Can the cancer spread while I am being treated with chemotherapy?
A:

Q: How can I tell if the cancer is coming back? Are there any danger signs to look out for?
A:

Q: Are there any foods I should or should not take during treatment? What about alcohol? Smoking? Supplements or vitamins?
A:

Q: Are there any exercises I should do or avoid during treatment?
A:

QUESTIONS for...

MY MEDICAL ONCOLOGIST (cont'd.)

Dr. _____ Date (mmddyyyy) _____

DURING OR FOLLOWING CHEMOTHERAPY

Q: Can you tell me how I am progressing? Am I doing OK, better or worse than you might expect?
A:

THE FOLLOWING THINGS CONCERN ME:

Q: I am experiencing **pain** (describe) _____ in these areas _____
    Are unusual sensations and/or pain normal during treatment? Why? What can I do to lessen it?
A:

Q: I am on these **medications** _____
    _____
    _____
    Will taking additional medication be safe or interfere with the ones I am already on?
A:

Q: I am experiencing these **side effects** _____
    Is this normal during treatment? Why? What can I do to lessen them?
A:

ABOUT BLOOD WORK

Q: Are you tracking a specific tumor marker in my case? If so, what is it? What is considered normal?
    What is mine? Are you satisfied with the results?
A:

Q: How often will I have blood and tumor marker tests?
A:

Q: What is my red blood count (HGB)? What is normal? How does mine compare with normal?
A:

Q: What is my white blood count (WGB)? What is normal? How does mine compare with normal?
A:

Remember to ask for copies of test results before you leave the office.

QUESTIONS
for...

MY RADIATION ONCOLOGIST

Dr. _____ Date (mmddyyyy) _____

BEFORE

Q: Why are you suggesting this test? (Eg. MRI, X-ray, CT scan or PET scan)
A:

Q: Who will administer this test, and where?
A:

Q: Please describe what the procedure will entail? (Length of time, requirement to be immobile etc.)
A:

Q: Do I need to fast before this test? For how long?
A:

Q: How soon will I get the results?
A:

AFTER

Q: Do the test results give you additional information? If so, what?
A:

Q: Does it show improvement?
A:

Q: If not, what is the next step?
A:

Q: Do you recommend any other testing or a new treatment? If so, what and why?
A:

QUESTIONS
for...

MY COMPLEMENTARY, ALTERNATIVE
AND INTEGRATIVE PRACTITIONERS

Dr. _____ Date (mmddyyyy) _____

Tell the specialist or practitioner clearly why you are seeking help:

☐ To complement your conventional physicians,

☐ For a general consultation

☐ Specifically for pain management or nausea

☐ For an alternative approach, complete in itself.

Check above or add your reason here:

_____

Q: What can I expect from your approach?
A:

Q: How much experience have you had with cancer patients and specifically with my kind of cancer and my kind of conventional treatments?
A:

Q: Are you willing to work with conventional doctors?
A:

Q: What is the knowledge base for the treatment you are recommending? Specifically, are there any published data for this treatment?
A:

Q: Are there any potential downsides?
A:

Q: What is the length of treatment?
A:

Q: If you are suggesting vitamins and supplements please specify brand names you know to be trustworthy and tell me why you are recommending them.
A:

Q: How will your suggestions for diet, whole food and supplements affect my conventional treatment?
A:

Q: What out-of-pocket costs will be involved? Fees for each visit? For supplements, etc?
A:

OTHER ADVANCE PREPARATION

❀ Mark all your appointments on a weekly or monthly calendar—paper or electronic, noting time, place, and practitioner. **Keep this calendar even *after* your appointments to verify your billing when it comes in.**

❀ Find out well ahead of time whether your doctor requires you to fill out any forms prior to your visit and whether he / she has access to your electronic records. If not, provide any contact information necessary for a smooth transmission of vital information from another office and make sure to follow up as appropriate. Without your records, your doctor, or a medical specialist, may not be able to assess your situation properly.

❀ If your appointment is for a test, make sure you understand any pre-consultation instructions such as dietary restrictions.

A FEW PRETTY GOOD TIPS

FOR MY NEXT APPOINTMENT

Use the pocket inside the front cover of your binder as a temporary holding place where you can keep a folder for the papers you will need for an upcoming appointment.

Before each visit

❀ Ask yourself "What papers do I need to take with me?" These may include previous tests and reports you may need to refer to at your appointment.

❀ Select your reports, notes, questions for the practitioner, etc. Before you move them, pencil on them where they belong so that you can return them to the correct place.

❀ Place a sticky note as a page marker at the original location before moving any papers.

❀ Transfer your selected information to this pocket. For a second opinion consultation, it is likely that you will need most, or all, of your medical information. For follow-up visits with your regular doctor, you will need much less, especially if you have given him or her permission to make copies.

❀ Take your updated *My Yellow Pages* (especially your Emergency Contact Numbers and Chronological Health Log) to all your appointments.

After each visit

❀ Return the papers to their original location unless you need them for your next appointment.

ON APPOINTMENT DAYS

BEFORE YOU LEAVE HOME

Be sure to bring the papers you have prepared for your next appointment with you.

❀ Check if a support person is allowed to accompany you into the medical building. If so, plan accordingly and meet the family member, friend or local oncology group representative early enough to share your list of questions and talk together about the purpose of your visit, and the kind of support you would appreciate (if you have not already done so).

❀ Call the office beforehand to find out if the doctor is on schedule, or your appointment will be delayed due to an emergency. This is not unusual. You might be able to adjust your schedule.

❀ If you wish to record your visit, take a small recording device, ready for that possibility.

❀ Think about how best to take care of yourself while waiting. For example, choose a good book, magazine or bring along a portable music player with ear phones. You might also want a bottle of water and a shawl cover-up for the cold examining rooms.

❀ Remember to bring your mask to wear indoors, if still mandated.

IN THE WAITING ROOM OR FRONT OFFICE

❀ On arrival, be friendly to the person at the front desk, and make a note of his or her name. A receptionist can be a helpful ally when you are making future appointments or when you have practical questions to ask. Introduce your companion. Confirm that you have permission for him/her to be present during the consultation.

❀ Relax with some deep breaths and feel your feet firmly on the ground.

❀ Ask the person accompanying you to be prepared to take notes for you and remind him or her of what you particularly wish the focus to be.

❀ Add any last minute questions to your list that arise while you are waiting.

❀ If something is bothering you, such as a noisy TV or insufficient ventilation, and you are really uncomfortable, ask the office receptionist if there's a way to remedy the situation.

❀ Check if the doctor is going to be delayed. If so, consider a walk or wait in your car, the hospital cafeteria or a local cafe. Check back just before the anticipated adjusted time or, before you leave the waiting room, request that the receptionist call your cell phone when the health professional is almost ready to see you.

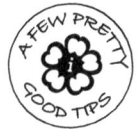

A FEW PRETTY GOOD TIPS

DURING YOUR CONSULTATION
OR DURING A TELEMEDICINE VISIT.*

Any reference to a companion assumes that you will follow current guidelines.

INITIAL CONNECTIONS AND QUESTIONS

* If your anxiety level is high, when entering the office, remind yourself that that you have prepared well and have your list of questions with you, and the person accompanying you is there to support you. Even if you don't always hear or remember everything that is being said, your companion will catch things you might miss. Ask your companion to write the answers to your questions so you can keep breathing—and stay present.

* Ask the physician for permission to record the consultation, especially if a support person is not allowed to be with you..

* Listen to what the doctor has to say. Note any questions that arise while you are listening and ask your companion to check off those that have been addressed. Ask for clarification whenever you feel you need it.

* Go through your list of questions and ask all of them systematically.

* If you feel rushed, breathe deeply again and ask the health practitioner to slow down. Ask your companion if she / he understands the gist of what is being said, and to rephrase the answer back to you to make sure you understand it.

* Feeling that you are interviewing your doctor may also boost your confidence. Your questions are NOT an imposition on your health providers. Questions help practitioners to know more about you, so that they can do a better job.

* If your physician doesn't appear to be listening to you or is not willing to answer your questions, that person may not be the best professional for you.

* **Do *not* sign up for treatment on the spot. You need time to integrate what you have heard before you come to a decision.**

***TELEMEDICINE / TELEONCOLOGY** is helpful IF you are not able to visit your doctor. It enables the remote diagnosis, treatment and follow-up of patients by means of telecommunications technology, using HIPPA compliant video-conferencing tools.

MEDICAL VISIT WORKSHEET

Some medical offices provide a printout of a "Clinical Visit Summary of Today's Visit". If not, use this form.

Visit to _____ Reason for visit _____

Initial routine check-in with _____

Vital signs: Weight _____   Temperature: _____ Blood pressure _____

Pulse: _____   Blood count _____   Other _____

Meeting with _____ MD

Nurse Practitioner/ Specialist / Other _____

My update (since last diagnosis) _____

_____

Comments in response _____

_____

My concerns _____

_____

Comments in response _____

_____

My questions _____

_____

_____

Answers given _____

_____

_____

Follow up suggestions / next steps _____

_____

_____

_____

NOTES

PART 4

FOLLOWING UP AFTER APPOINTMENTS

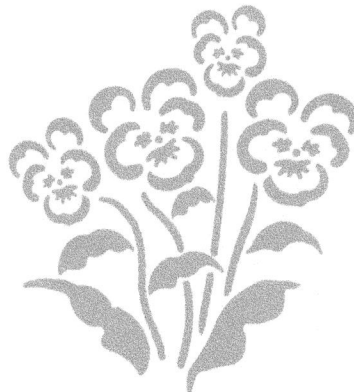

AFTER MY MEDICAL APPOINTMENTS
Organize your notes while your memory is still fresh.

SUMMARIZE YOUR PRIORITIES **on the next page after every health care visit whether at a conventional or complementary practitioner's office or at a hospital.**

❃ Identify each meeting clearly with the medical professional's name and the date.

❃ Note any matters that you want to follow-up—further research, reading, or interviews. Include your personal observations and impressions. Add self-care (non-medical) ideas that you might also wish to explore.

❃ Update any decisions.

Update your medical history in your *Chronological Health & Cancer Log* after every visit. It will become a useful reference for all your practitioners, as well as for yourself.

Make a note of your next appointment in your calendar.

Complete your *Review and Update Medical Healthcare Progress* (on pages 58–59) on a regular basis. As you review your progress, renew your commitment to good health. Remind yourself that your health is in your hands as well as your doctor's. You can use your mind, emotions, and spirit to help your body heal.

A FEW PRETTY GOOD TIPS

GETTING THE ANSWERS YOU NEED

❃ **Review with your companion your Q. and A. notes of what was said and the course of action suggested by the professional, *as soon after your appointment as possible.*** Details can fade very fast, especially if you did not record the appointment. Underline the important points the doctor made about your diagnosis, his or her answers, and recommendations. If you are not sure about any aspect of the discussion or if your perceptions differ greatly from those of the person accompanying you, identify the area of confusion and reframe a question to clarify it.

❃ Consider sending these subsequent questions to your doctor's office for attention. If your writing is very difficult to read, type or ask someone to type key information / questions.

❃ If you come away from an appointment sensing your questions were not being addressed, or you are not clear about an explanation, don't consider your lack of understanding as unintelligent or your doubts as silly. Honor them as contributing to your well-being—and note questions you now wish to ask. If necessary, talk to someone from an oncology support group or cancer chatroom who understands medical implications / terminology.

SUMMARIZE PRIORITIES AFTER EVERY HEALTHCARE VISIT

Dr. ______________________________ Date (mmddyyyy) ____________

Preferred way to be contacted: ______________________________

MY DOCTOR'S, OR OTHER PROFESSIONAL'S, MOST IMPORTANT RECOMMENDATIONS

To do now:

"Down the line" recommendations for later:

MY RESPONSE

After reviewing my experience and my notes, THE MOST IMPORTANT OUTCOMES of this appointment are: ______________________________

____

My predominant feelings are: ______________________________

____

Follow-up actions I might take:

Schedule an additional test? YES / NO

Get a second opinion / see another practitioner? YES / NO

Schedule a recommended treatment? For what? ______________ When? __________

Explore further research? YES / NO

Check out other resources recommended? YES / NO

Postpone any follow-up until I have further information or additional test results? YES / NO

Do I need more information about technical / medical words, procedures, etc. that I don't fully understand? YES / NO

IF YES to any questions, note when and how to follow up...

My impressions of the practitioner, staff and the facility:

Strengths? E.g. welcoming, friendly, professional, knowledgeable? ______________

Practitioner's capacity to listen and communicate answers to my questions clearly? ______________

Other? ______________________________

Weaknesses? E.g. preoccupied or impatient staff; stuffy or noisy facility? ______________

Other? ______________________________

Do I wish to continue with this professional? YES / NO

REVIEW AND UPDATE MEDICAL HEALTHCARE PROGRESS

Weekly, monthly or whenever you wish to take an inventory of your progress.

Reviewing your medical healthcare progress after a number of visits will give you an overview of a bigger picture and you will notice if anything is falling through the cracks.

FOR THE PERIOD FROM _____ TO _____

What are the most significant ideas to have emerged from consultations / conversations?

How might I follow-up these ideas?

PROGRESS

Is there an overall treatment plan in place?

- If not, who can help me put one in place?

- If so, how is this plan progressing?

- What specific progress has been made since my last review?

Is my treatment plan proceeding in a timely manner?

- Do I feel rushed to make decisions?

- Am I satisfied with the rate of progress?

REVIEW & UPDATE MEDICAL HEALTHCARE PROGRESS (Cont'd)

COMMUNICATION

⊱ Am I being kept informed? Am I sufficiently included in the decision-making loop?

• Have reports been sent to the practitioners I have so requested?

• Are my health care providers communicating about, and coordinating, my treatment?

• If not, where specifically is coordination lacking?

CURRENT TREATMENT GOALS FROM _____ UNTIL _____

⊱ What are my treatment goals?

• For next week? Beginning date _____

• Next month? Beginning date _____

• Three months hence? From_____ to _____

OTHER OBSERVATIONS

⊱ How do I feel?

• How is my body responding to treatment?

• Am I experiencing any fatigue, aches, pains, unusual body sensations or any differences in my sleep pattern?

Check often that your treatment log is fully up-to-date and that you have noted all upcoming appointments in your calendar.

When you review your medical health care progress, take a moment to review your self-care progress also.

ORGANIZE DOCTORS' PAPERWORK

Identify all your currently active doctors and health care practitioners.

Your active team might include your primary care physician, gynecologist, healer, oncologist, nutritionist, radiologist, surgeon, acupuncturist, naturopath, and massage therapist.

Organize each practitioner's papers separately.

Arrange each set of papers in dated order, with the most recent report on top.

Remember to add the date mm/dd/**yyyy**. (Especially the year).

For each, include records of all consultations or visits, your preparatory questions, doctors' answers, your follow-up notes, and prescriptions or recommendations you receive.

Create a tab divider for each practitioner and arrange them in alphabetical order or whatever way works for you.

A FEW PRETTY GOOD TIPS

SO MANY DOCTORS, SO MANY TABS

You may be surprised at the number of specialists you may be asked to consult, and in addition, you may have complementary care appointments. You don't need to use a separate tab for everyone in an office. (i.e. All paperwork with regard to your primary care physician, his or her nurse, physician's assistant, and receptionist would go in your primary care physician's section.)

If you are interested in, or are combining, both conventional medicine and complementary care, divide your information into two parts: one for conventional and another for complementary. If you are seeing an integrative doctor, keep both parts together.

If you have enrolled in any Online Patient Portals, keep a clear record of its name and the information you can access, along with your password for each.

Note: Do not include financial or legal papers along with your medical papers. It is more efficient to keep them separately; perhaps in another secure place.

ORGANIZE TESTS, REPORTS AND MEDICATIONS

Identify tests you have had such as blood work, lab results, pathology and consultation records; and ask your doctor or hospital to provide copies of results once they are available.

Fill out the pages for:

Results from laboratories and other facilities

Medications, pharmacies and other suppliers

Vitamins, minerals, supplements and suppliers

Put medical reports and test results from each type of test together with your notes, in dated order, most recent on top, and file them behind the appropriate divider.

For example, keep radiology and blood work reports separate from each other within this section. It will then be easier to reference them at your next visit or set of tests.

FILING YOUR REPORTS

In the beginning it may not seem necessary to separate the reports, but later it becomes essential as more and more information will come your way.

❀ Highlight the date of test results or lab-work mm/dd/**yyyy** (Remember the year).

❀ Add notes you have made related to going for tests and receiving results.

Keep medical release forms and privacy statements connected to these tests with your legal records.

*The use of "certified" **Electronic Health Records (EHRs)** is almost universally in place in hospitals and physicians' offices, so that patient records can be easily transmitted as needed. Since 2016 all health care providers are required to make electronic copies of patient records available to patients, at their request, in machine-readable form. (The 21st Century Cures Act.).

In this digital age, it is highly unlikely that you will be asked to transport your records from one doctor to another for an upcoming appt.

RESULTS FROM LABORATORIES AND OTHER FACILITIES GIVING REPORTS

Name of lab or facility _____

Contact person _____

Address _____

Tel _____ Fax _____ Email _____

Best way to contact _____

TEST _____

Date (mmddyyyy) _____

Reason _____

Results _____

Filed?   Yes / No

Name of lab or facility _____

Contact person _____

Address _____

Tel _____ Fax _____ Email _____

Best way to contact _____

TEST _____

Date _____

Reason _____

Results _____

Filed?   Yes / No

Name of lab or facility _____

Contact person _____

Address _____

Tel _____ Fax _____ Email _____

Best way to contact _____

TEST _____

Date _____

Reason _____

Results _____

Filed?   Yes / No

Name of lab or facility _____

Contact person _____

Address _____

Tel _____ Fax _____ Email _____

Best way to contact _____

TEST _____

Date _____

Reason _____

Results _____

Filed?   Yes / No

Name of lab or facility _____

Contact person _____

Address _____

Tel _____ Fax _____ Email _____

Best way to contact _____

TEST _____

Date _____

Reason _____

Results _____

Filed?   Yes / No

Name of lab or facility _____

Contact person _____

Address _____

Tel _____ Fax _____ Email _____

Best way to contact _____

TEST _____

Date _____

Reason _____

Results _____

Filed?   Yes / No

MEDICATION AND PHARMACIES / SUPPLIERS

For each medication note the following information:

Name of medication _____ Circle: generic / brand | **Pharmacy or Supplier:**

Prescribed by_____ Date **(mmddyyyy)**_____ | _____

For_____Dosage _____ | Contact person _____

Date began _____Instructions _____ | Address _____

Doctors informed of new prescription _____ | Best way to contact: _____

Positive/negative results/side effects _____ | _____

Name of medication _____ Circle: generic / brand | **Pharmacy or Supplier:**

Prescribed by_____ Date _____ | _____

For_____Dosage _____ | Contact person _____

Date began _____Instructions _____ | Address _____

Doctors informed of new prescription _____ | Best way to contact: _____

Positive/negative results/side effects _____ | _____

Name of medication _____ Circle: generic / brand | **Pharmacy or Supplier:**

Prescribed by_____ Date _____ | _____

For_____Dosage _____ | Contact person _____

Date began _____Instructions _____ | Address _____

Doctors informed of new prescription _____ | Best way to contact: _____

Positive/negative results/side effects _____ | _____

Name of medication _____ Circle: generic / brand | **Pharmacy or Supplier:**

Prescribed by_____ Date _____ | _____

For_____Dosage _____ | Contact person _____

Date began _____Instructions _____ | Address _____

Doctors informed of new prescription _____ | Best way to contact: _____

Positive/negative results/side effects _____ | _____

Name of medication _____ Circle: generic / brand | **Pharmacy or Supplier:**

Prescribed by_____ Date _____ | _____

For_____Dosage _____ | Contact person _____

Date began _____Instructions _____ | Address _____

Doctors informed of new prescription _____ | Best way to contact: _____

Positive/negative results/side effects _____ | _____

VITAMINS, MINERALS, SUPPLEMENTS AND SUPPLIERS

For each vitamin, mineral or supplement, note the following information:

Name of vitamin/supplement _____   **Manufacturer** _____

Authorized by _____ Date (mmddyyyy) _____   **Source of supply:**

For _____ Dosage _____   Health Food Store_____

Date began _____ Instructions _____   Pharmacy _____

Doctors/practitioners informed of supplement _____   Online _____

Positive/negative results/side effects _____   _____

Name of vitamin/supplement _____   **Manufacturer** _____

Authorized by _____ Date _____   **Source of supply:**

For _____ Dosage _____   Health Food Store_____

Date began _____ Instructions _____   Pharmacy _____

Doctors/practitioners informed of supplement _____   Online _____

Positive/negative results/side effects _____   _____

Name of vitamin/supplement _____   **Manufacturer** _____

Authorized by _____ Date _____   **Source of supply:**

For _____ Dosage _____   Health Food Store_____

Date began _____ Instructions _____   Pharmacy _____

Doctors/practitioners informed of supplement _____   Online _____

Positive/negative results/side effects _____   _____

Name of vitamin/supplement _____   **Manufacturer** _____

Authorized by _____ Date _____   **Source of supply:**

For _____ Dosage _____   Health Food Store_____

Date began _____ Instructions _____   Pharmacy _____

Doctors/practitioners informed of supplement _____   Online _____

Positive/negative results/side effects _____   _____

Name of vitamin/supplement _____   **Manufacturer** _____

Authorized by _____ Date _____   **Source of supply:**

For _____ Dosage _____   Health Food Store_____

Date began _____ Instructions _____   Pharmacy _____

Doctors/practitioners informed of supplement _____   Online _____

Positive/negative results/side effects _____   _____

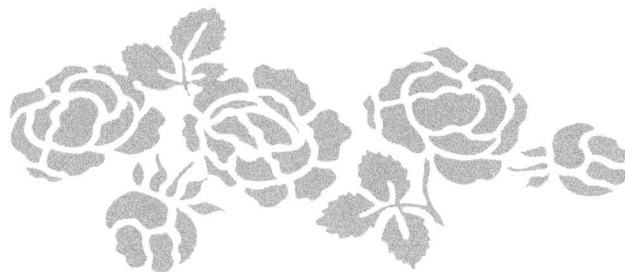

PART 5

BILLS, INSURANCE AND LEGAL RECORDS

ORGANIZE BILLS

It is highly unlikely that you will need to brings any papers pertaining to billing to your medical appointments. Consider keeping all your financial papers, including bills in clearly marked folders in a drawer of a filing cabinet or in a firebox. Keep them separate from other medical notes pertaining to health practitioners or test results. If you do wish to keep them in a separate binder, use divider tabs and clear sheet protectors or pockets.

MAKE AND RECORD PAYMENTS

First, separate out UNPAID bills and PAID bills.

UNPAID BILLS (PENDING):

Put all your unpaid bills in the *UNPAID BILLS* section until they have been paid and acknowledged as paid. Review regularly.

Place an urgent bill in a special section or folder earmarked for that purpose with a name such as "IMMEDIATE ATTENTION," and keep it in an obvious place where you cannot forget it. Then take action as soon as you can.

Keep doctors' bills together with insurance bills if you have health insurance, since health providers and insurance companies are closely connected through billing practices.

And especially separate out UNPAID BILLS from PAID BILLS if you and your insurance are each paying a portion.

PAID BILLS:

Use the *PAID BILLS* section when NO further payment is required in connection with the charge. As your bills are completed and accumulate, consider transferring them to a separate folder/binder marked "Completed" as you don't need to take them to appointments.

DIVIDE YOUR PAID BILLS into the following 3 categories behind the appropriate dividers:

1. **Non-reimbursable Bills**—You alone are responsible for paying these bills.

2. **Reimbursable Bills (Primary Insurance)** You expect your primary insurance company to pay in part or in whole.

   File here only those primary insurance bills that require *no* further payment in connection with the charge.

   Put these bills together in dated order, most recent on top.

3. **Reimbursable Bills (Secondary Insurance)** You expect your secondary insurance company to pay in part or in whole.

   File your secondary insurance bills when it is clear that *no* further payment is required in connection with the charge.

   Put these bills together in dated order, most recent on top.

PAYING BILLS

⊛ **Check thoroughly before you pay any bill.** Sometimes statements are very confusing and often arrive quite a long time after your actual appointment. Some charges are even incorrect. Refer to your medical calendar to check that the date on the bill corresponds to the date of the appointment.

⊛ **Make a copy of the bill and file it before paying.** Note on the bill the date on which you paid it, the check number, and the name of any person you spoke to in connection with the payment.

⊛ **A**sk for help if you are not confident about interpreting bills—contact the person in the billing department of your physician's office, or a social worker.

⊛ **Keep accurate copies of all medical bills, insurance statements (often called Explanation of Benefits or EOB's) and receipts.** This will serve you well when it's tax time.

TAX DEDUCTIONS

❀ Ask a tax preparer or financial adviser about tax deductions in connection with your illness, and the information they will need from you.

❀ Keep a monthly tally of all your expenses as follows. (It will be easier at the end of the year):

Monthly

Premium payments	$ _____
Travel expenses	$ _____
Co-pay	$ _____
Co-insurance	$ _____
Prescriptions	$ _____
Total	$ _____

Annual

Total premium payments	$ _____
Total travel expenses	$ _____
Total co-pay	$ _____
Total co-insurance	$ _____
Total prescriptions	$ _____
Annual insurance deductible	$ _____
Total	$ _____

❀ Subtract any payments reimbursed by your insurance company, as you will not be able to claim them.

❀ Keep an accurate record of all your medical expenses for the IRS in order to claim them on your tax return. Note mileage and keep all gas, toll, hotel, meal, rail, bus and airline receipts for every health related journey, as well as other out-of-pocket expenses such as prescription drugs and medical equipment.

ORGANIZE INSURANCE CLAIMS AND RECORDS

USE THE *WHAT MY INSURANCE COVERS* FORM (page 74) to clarify exactly what you can expect from your Insurance Company or include a copy of your policy in your binder.

FILL OUT *MY CONTACTS WITH INSURANCE COMPANIES* FORM (page 71), to record all contacts with your insurance company, including calls, emails and letters. Attach copies of any correspondence or forms submitted.

Enter your insurance information, including membership I.D., plan name and policy numbers for all your insurance carriers, in your Yellow Pages.

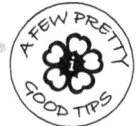

KNOW YOUR POLICY

Review your policy/policies carefully, *before* you get any treatment. Annual deductibles, co-payments per office visit, test, prescription drugs (brand name and generic), ambulance service, or wellness care allowed can vary greatly.

Many different types of health plans exist, including group plans, individual plans, HMO's, disability income insurance, long-term care plans, Medicaid, and for seniors—Medicare. There are now specific personal *cancer* indemnity plans in some states. An HMO policy requires you to choose a local participating doctor or facility, or pay out of pocket non-reimbursable expenses for services outside your network plan.

The right kind of coverage should provide benefits for in-patient hospital care, physician services, lab work and X-rays, prescription drugs, outpatient services and nursing home care at a location of your choice. If necessary, get help from your insurance provider to understand your plan.

A FEW PRETTY GOOD TIPS

WHAT MY INSURANCE COVERS (PRIMARY AND SUPPLEMENTARY)

My outpatient benefits are:

My inpatient benefits are:

What are the different co-payments or percentage co-insurance I have to make for

Inpatient _____   Specialist _____

Outpatient_____   Mental health practitioner _____

Primary care physician _____   My annual deductible _____

What % do I have to pay after my annual deductible is met?_____

What is the maximum life-time benefit / cap, if any? _____

How do I file a claim?

Do I have out-of-network benefits? If so, what is the co-pay? _____

Will my insurance cover the following?

Second opinions?   YES / NO   Home healthcare?   YES / NO

Clinical trials?   YES / NO   Other _____ ?   YES / NO

If yes, do I need a referral, and from whom? _____

When must I get preauthorization for treatment or consultations? _____

If pre-authorization is required, who has to make the treatment referral? _____

MY CONTACTS WITH INSURANCE COMPANIES

To / From: _____(Person contacted) **Insurance company** _____

   Tel. #_____ Ext._____

   Date(mmddyyyy) _____ Time _____ **Claim / reference number** _____

Question, issue or dispute discussed _____

   Answer/action needed/ agreed _____

To / From: _____(Person contacted) **Insurance company** _____

   Tel. #_____ Ext._____

   Date _____ Time _____ **Claim / reference number** _____

Question, issue or dispute discussed _____

   Answer/action needed/ agreed _____

To / From: _____(Person contacted) **Insurance company** _____

   Tel. #_____ Ext._____

   Date _____ Time _____ **Claim / reference number** _____

Question, issue or dispute discussed _____

   Answer/action needed/ agreed _____

To / From: _____(Person contacted) **Insurance company** _____

   Tel. #_____ Ext._____

   Date _____ Time _____ **Claim / reference number** _____

Question, issue or dispute discussed _____

   Answer/action needed/ agreed _____

To / From: _____(Person contacted) **Insurance company** _____

   Tel. #_____ Ext._____

   Date _____ Time _____ **Claim / reference number** _____

Question, issue or dispute discussed _____

   Answer/action needed/ agreed _____

SUBMITTING CLAIMS

At your first visit, expect health care providers to ask for and make a copy of your current insurance card(s) and your driver's license or State approved ID. Ask whether they will submit a claim on your behalf or whether you will have to do this yourself. If they agree to submit your claim, and you don't receive paperwork in a timely fashion, say three weeks, check in with them to make sure they have followed through.

If necessary, get help filing claims. Some insurance companies have case managers. In a situation where you are likely to have on-going contact with your insurer, ask if they will assign a case manager to you. That's not always possible, so if you find yourself talking to a particularly helpful representative, thank that person, **request his or her name and telephone extension,** and ask to be connected to that extension in future calls.

If you don't understand a bill or an Explanation of Benefits or if the amount is different from what you expect, keep asking questions. **Insurance companies can make mistakes. Be persistent.**

If your insurance company rejects a claim that has been submitted, call the company to ask their representative why it was rejected. Then immediately call the billing person in your medical professional's office. Explain what the insurance representative told you and ask them to look into the matter on your behalf. If you are still not satisfied, don't give up—file again. A wrong code for your diagnosis is a common error. Other reasons a claim is denied include a decision that your procedure was not medically necessary, that you have a pre-existing condition, that it is a "non-covered" benefit or that you have chosen to go "out-of-network."

If a claim you still understand to be justified is again rejected, request the insurance company's appeal process and make an appeal. Ask someone to review your letter before you send it in to make sure it is clear and accurate.

If you feel that the insurance company is inappropriately handling your case, or if you have a continuing unresolved dispute, lodge a complaint with your state's Insurance Department. You may be able to do this online. For example, New York State residents can go to www.ins.state.ny.us. A local Legal Aid office might also help.

Don't get discouraged.
Take a break, go for a walk, have a cup of tea, call up a friend, ask for help and come back to it later.

ORGANIZE LEGAL PAPERS

Divide your legal records behind the dividers for CURRENT TREATMENT and FUTURE LIFE CHOICES.

* **CURRENT TREATMENT:** You will be asked to sign many different types of forms.

   Sub-divide the following as you receive them:
   * Consent forms for treatment
   * Medical release forms
   * Privacy statements
   * Other legal papers

* **DO NOT SIGN ANY CONSENT FORMS, if the exact procedure has not been described or if you do not understand it. Your consent must be fully informed.**
   Cross out statements that are not in agreement with your wishes. Even if your doctor has forceful opinions and strong recommendations, it is your decision and responsibility, as a mentally competent adult, to accept or refuse treatment.

   Consider keeping consent forms and medical release forms in a separate binder as you will rarely refer to them.

Consider keeping important papers in a fire-proof box.

* **FUTURE LIFE CHOICES: Advance directives** ensure your wishes are as binding as possible concerning end-of-life issues and what you wish to pass onto your loved ones. (See page 76 for details of legal and non-binding advance directives.)

   Make sure you fill out the following legal forms AS SOON AS POSSIBLE, if you have not already done so. This will make it easy for yourself and your loved ones at a later date:
   * Living Will*
   * Health Care Proxy* or Agent (health care power of attorney)
   * Will
   * Power of Attorney

   Search the Internet to download state-specific forms that will be honored as legal if properly signed.
   Note who has a copy of each in *My Yellow Pages*, once you have filled them out.

* When preparing your Living Will and your Healthcare Proxy, I highly recommend "FIVE WISHES," available from www.agingwithdignity.org 1-888-5-WISHES / 1-888-594-7437. The Five Wishes are for: "1. The person I want to make care decisions for me when I can't; 2. The kind of medical treatment I want or don't want; 3. How comfortable I want to be; 4. How I want people to treat me; and 5. What I want my loved ones to know."

LEGAL ADVANCE DIRECTIVES

These include

Health care proxy—delegating authority to another person to make health care decisions on your behalf, if you become mentally or physically incapacitated.

Living will—expressing your wishes, to guide your healthcare proxy, as to what your medical treatment should be. For example, you might wish to receive all possible medical interventions or you might refuse treatment that will artificially prolong your life. As previously stated, it's your right to decide to request or refuse treatment as a mentally competent adult.

Granting power of attorney—for non-health issues such as financial and other personal matters.

Writing a will or creating a trust— transferring your assets in accordance with your desires as opposed to your assets being transferred pursuant to state law.

It is wise to consult an attorney to ensure that any documents you have downloaded from the Internet **are in accordance with your state laws** and court precedents (not federal law).

❀ Give a copy of your living will to all significant family members, your doctors, your healthcare proxy and your lawyer. Make sure *everyone* knows about your decision to accept or decline treatment that will artificially prolong your life. It simply isn't enough to sign a living will and have it filed away.

❀ List where you keep these important documents in *My Yellow Pages*, Page 13.

Preparing advance directives does not mean you are about to die. Life will be much easier for your beloved family and friends if they know your wishes.

NON-BINDING ADVANCE DIRECTIVES

Prepare non-binding advance directives at your leisure such as:

❀ Ethical Will (heartfelt thoughts, passing on your love and beliefs to family member and friends)

❀ Other papers (letters or gifts to specific individuals.)

PART 6

MY REFERENCE LIBRARY

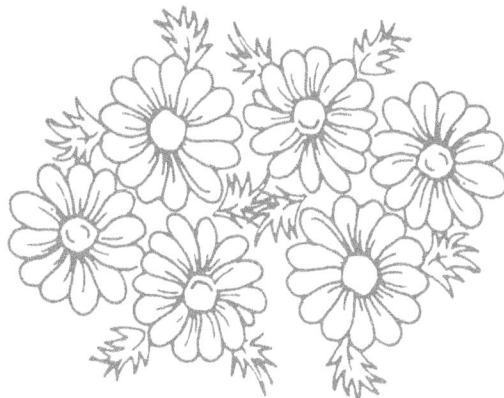

RESOURCES AND INFORMATION

Start to collect resources *at your own pace*.

Your resources might include information about:
- Organizations (health / community etc), internet and websites, newsletters and magazines
- Books, audios and videos, consulting, treatment information and referral services
- Research reports and cancer articles, internet search engines, sources and information
- Sources of less expensive vitamins, organic produce, drugs
- Humor: movies, cartoons
- Personal anecdotes and miscellaneous resources

Use the organizing pages and tabs to divide information as best suits you.
- People and organizations to contact
- Good ideas from conversations / emails
- Suggestions to remember
- Favorite resources

A FEW PRETTY GOOD TIPS

There is a lot of information out there in all shapes and sizes, especially on the internet. It can be overpowering and possibly incorrect. If you are a person who is reassured by having a lot of information, you will be comfortable gathering it. Helpful guidelines for evaluating websites can be found at http://medlineplus.gov/healthywebsurfing.html

Initially, you'll be able to put the material at the back of your organizer. Quite soon, you may find it necessary to sort it according to topic and place it in folders, file boxes or filing cabinet drawers.

If you are easily overwhelmed by lots of facts and figures, delegate this task to someone else.

PEOPLE AND ORGANIZATIONS TO CONTACT

List each person or organization you've heard about, and might like to contact at some point.

Name_____

Organization _____

Address (if known) _____

Tel/email/web site (if known) _____

Reason for contacting_____

Where I found out about this_____

Name_____

Organization _____

Address (if known) _____

Tel/email/web site (if known) _____

Reason for contacting_____

Where I found out about this_____

Name_____

Organization _____

Address (if known) _____

Tel/email/web site (if known) _____

Reason for contacting_____

Where I found out about this_____

Name_____

Organization _____

Address (if known) _____

Tel/email/web site (if known) _____

Reason for contacting_____

Where I found out about this_____

Name_____

Organization _____

Address (if known) _____

Tel/email/web site (if known) _____

Reason for contacting_____

Where I found out about this_____

GOOD IDEAS FROM CONVERSATIONS AND EMAILS

If you receive a helpful email, print it out and insert it with your resources / information.

Contact with (name of person) _____ On (date) _____

We discussed _____

New ideas / significant information _____

_____

I'll follow-up by _____

Contact with (name of person) _____ On (date) _____

We discussed _____

New ideas / significant information _____

_____

I'll follow-up by _____

Contact with (name of person) _____ On (date) _____

We discussed _____

New ideas / significant information _____

_____

I'll follow-up by _____

Contact with (name of person) _____ On (date) _____

We discussed _____

New ideas / significant information _____

_____

I'll follow-up by _____

Contact with (name of person) _____ On (date) _____

We discussed _____

New ideas / significant information _____

_____

I'll follow-up by _____

FAVORITE RESOURCES

If you use a computer for record keeping, note where this information is stored.

Articles

Books / Ebooks

Magazines

FAVORITE RESOURCES (cont'd)

Web sites

Advocacy Organizations

National Organizations

Other—such as Medical Research Organizations

Local or Hospital Libraries

Blogs

PART 7

MY SURVIVORSHIP WELLNESS PLAN

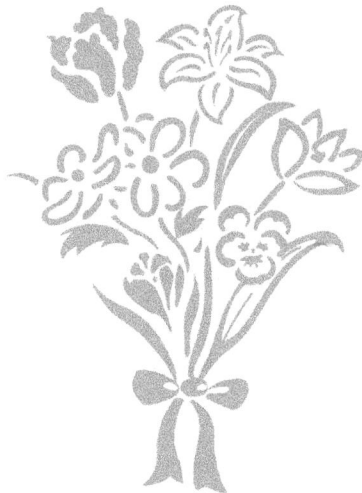

PLANNING FOR SURVIVORSHIP

When your treatment ends, you may have mixed feelings about what lies ahead. You may feel happy and relieved that your medical visits need not be frequent, yet you may be somewhat apprehensive without the monitoring and encouragement that regular visits to a trusted health professional have given you. A survivorship plan is intended to support and guide you. Cancer physicians and cancer facilities are now required to provide a written post-treatment care plan to discuss with you. Addressing your future health concerns and care with your doctor's plan in hand will hopefully alleviate any sense you may have of being vulnerable, without an anchor, as you move forward.

Before terminating treatment, expect your cancer doctor(s) to schedule an appointment to:

> ✑ Review your past treatment with you

and

> ✑ Offer written recommendations to form the basis of a comprehensive after-care survivorship plan.

If your doctors haven't offered their recommendations or encouraged you to make such a plan, it is never too late for you to initiate a conversation with them. You can use the guidelines below to prepare to put a plan in place.

It is vitally important that you are involved in creating your plan along with your cancer physician or other professionals who have been responsible for your treatment.

When you have agreed to—and have confidence—in your plan, you will be able to follow through whole-heartedly. That's *your* responsibility. It's *your* life!

OVERVIEW

> ✑ Your survivorship plan will outline key components of *where you have been* in your cancer treatment from beginning to end. Thus, you will have essential information at your fingertips to give to other doctors who may ask you about your cancer history.

> ✑ It will provide recommendations for your future care to guide your progress both to prevent a recurrence and to support you towards *where you want to go* to maintain good health. It will include information about who is best to contact when you have medical questions, what further tests may be needed, the frequency of visits, and how to maintain your health with regular exercise, a healthy diet, and emotional and spiritual support that will work for you.

HOW TO SET UP YOUR PLAN

STEP 1: DECIDE WHO WILL HELP YOU

Ask yourself:

- Are any of the doctors who have been professionally involved in my cancer care required to contribute to my post-treatment plan by reviewing my treatment and making recommendations?

  If so, please name:

  - Medical oncologist _____

  - Surgeon _____

  - Radiation oncologist _____

  - Other _____

  - Note if one of the above has already coordinated your treatment _____

- Are there other health-care practitioners whom I would like to contribute to my after-care plan?

  If so, please name:

  - Primary care physician / family doctor _____

  - Complementary or alternative practitioner _____

  - Social worker or mental health counselor _____

  - Other specialist _____

- Who would be the best or most appropriate person to *coordinate* my after-care plan?

  _____

- Is there a family member or close friend whose insights and help I would value for this project?

  _____

Note here those you would like to be involved:

Name	Date Invited	Date agreed/declined

STEP 2: WHERE I HAVE BEEN (MY TREATMENT HISTORY)

1 Ask your doctor to provide (if he/she has not done so) a written outline of the most important aspects of your treatment that would be essential information for future practitioners. Expect it to cover your:

Cancer diagnosis/diagnoses _____

Tests _____

Cancer treatment history with dates, location and physicians, such as:

Surgery—including your final pathology report after surgery, with the cancer stage and characteristics of the tumor _____

Chemotherapy—including type of chemo used _____

Hormone therapy _____

Immunotherapy _____

Radiation _____

Other treatments and doses _____

Side effects—of treatment, if any _____

Medication and doses _____

Side effects—of medicines/drugs, if any _____

Side effects—possible long-term side effects of any intervention _____

Clinical trials _____

For all of the above, and especially for any radiation therapy and chemotherapy, please indicate the beginning and ending dates with mm/dd/yyyy. You'd be surprised how easy it is to forget this information.

2 Review the information you gathered when you created a record of your cancer care in Parts 1–4. Make your own summary of what has been important to you on your cancer journey. Add it to your binder.

- Formulate a question for your doctor if you find anything you don't understand, and add it to your summary.

- Note where you can find more detailed information in your binder should you need it.

3 If you have not yet gathered all of your information in one place, follow the guidelines on pages 2, 60 and 61 to fill out, sort and transfer relevant paperwork regarding past treatments, test results, and medications etc. into the appropriate sections of a binder.

Your binder will then be helpful both to you and to your health professionals if you develop health issues later in life or change your physician or residence. It is likely that you will be asked the same set of questions again. Keep your binder safely in a place where you (or a family member) can easily retrieve it. You will have the information at your fingertips, especially if your records get lost or destroyed.

Be sure to bring your treatment summary to all future appointments.

STEP 3: WHERE I AM GOING (FUTURE CARE POSSIBILITIES)

1 Expect your doctor to provide:

- A written summary of FUTURE MEDICAL CARE RECOMMENDATIONS which will include your medical care team, a schedule for future medical visits, follow-up tests and appointments, noting to whom, frequency and location.

- A written summary of LIFESTYLE CHANGES RECOMMENDATIONS - healthy habits to prevent a recurrence and maintain general health and wellness.

2 List YOUR top priorities, hopes, needs, and intentions for your future health and well-being.

- Share these with your doctor and make sure they are reflected in your after-care treatment plan.

    1._____

    2._____

    3._____

    4._____

    5._____

- Remember to tap into your intuition and be prepared to share your perspectives with your doctor.

3 Review the list of possible questions below about your future medical care. Check those which are relevant to you and which you would like to discuss with your doctor:

🌱 Medical support:

Who will support / monitor me: my primary care physician, oncologist, other specialist or someone else?

When should I make an appointment to see:

My primary care physician? _____

My cancer doctor? _____

My surgeon? _____

Other specialists? _____

How often? _____

Under what circumstances? _____

If I am in pain?_____

If I have a particular problem, such as lymphedema? _____

If I continue to experience side effects of treatment or medication?_____

Other? _____

STEP 3: WHERE I AM GOING (FUTURE CARE POSSIBILITIES) (cont'd)

✥ Medical tests and screening:

How will I know if I need another test such as a Scan and X-ray, MRI, PET or CT Scan, lab test and/or blood-work? _____

Who will order the test?_____

Where do I go? _____

Who will give me the results and when? _____

What is the risk versus benefit ratio of any treatment or testing you have suggested? _____

_____

✥ Healthy lifestyle habits: *

• Diet

What foods will keep my immune system strong? _____

_____

What fruits and veggies are particularly healthy for cancer prevention? _____

_____

What should I avoid? _____

What about soy products? Dairy products? Red meat? _____

Alcohol, tobacco and sodas? _____

Weight—What is my ideal BMI (body mass index)? Have I any overweight / underweight issues?

_____

Other? _____

• Exercise

How frequently and for how long should I exercise? _____

Are there any exercises I would be better to avoid? _____

Other? _____

• Support to address emotional and/or spiritual concerns and needs

Are there any post-treatment survivorship groups? _____

_____

Can you recommend a therapist, emotional counselor or spiritual guide who has experience with cancer patients? _____

Other? _____

* Refer to what you have written on page 26. For detailed suggestions to bring balance to your body, mind, emotions and spirit, see Puja A. J. Thomson, After Shock: From Cancer Diagnosis to Healing, (Part 3 Reach In—Create Your Own Wellness Program: Pages 101-170).

STEP 3: WHERE I AM GOING (FUTURE CARE POSSIBILITIES) (cont'd)

༅ Risk factors

How can I lessen the risk of a recurrence? _____

_____

What known factors will negatively impact my overall health and increase the risk of a recurrence?

_____

4 **Note your non-medical concerns and those whom you might ask to help:**

Concern	Specific issue	Person(s) who can help
Aging		
Community resources		
Environmental toxicity		
Fears		
Health insurance		
Legal issues		
Long-term care		
Money		
Relationships		
Sexuality		
Spirituality		

STEP 4: AT YOUR SURVIVORSHIP WELLNESS APPOINTMENT

1 In advance, ask a family member, friend or navigator to accompany you to be another set of ears. You may also ask the doctor if you have permission to record the discussion. If he/she agrees, bring your own recording device with you.

2 When you meet your doctor, review his/her written recommendations. Make sure you question anything you don't understand, and that your top priorities for your future health and well-being have been taken into consideration.

3 Now you are ready to agree to your survivorship wellness plan.

STEP 5: AFTER YOUR SURVIVORSHIP WELLNESS APPOINTMENT

1 Confirm your willingness to commit to those aspects of your plan with which you and your doctor are in full agreement.

2 Prioritize and list those that are most important to you below:

MY SURVIVORSHIP WELLNESS PLAN AGREEMENT

To maintain my health and wellbeing, I commit to:	Now	Later

If you still have concerns or questions about other aspects of your plan, decide who will follow up—you, your doctor or someone else. Make a note of who will do what by when:

Concern/question	Person to follow-up	By (date)

STEP 6: NOW USE YOUR PLAN!

1 Put your updated agreed upon plan in your binder along with your doctor's treatment review and future recommendations.

2 Review your commitments regularly (monthly?) and renew, or change, as appropriate.

3 Keep your plan as up-to-date as possible and be sure to take it with you to any new appointments with your primary care doctor, gynecologist, oncology team and other specialists.

4 Use it to prepare for visits and to record any recommendations, as you did in Parts 1–4.

5 Expect your plan to grow over the years as your health changes. Be ready to add binders and/or subdivide your records so that you can still easily find the information when you need it.

AFTERWORD

Here's how it all began—as Barbara Sarah LCSW, Founder of the Health Alliance of the Hudson Valley Oncology Support Program, remembers:

Back when Puja Thomson and I were sitting in the waiting room of her breast surgeon's office in 2003 and I first saw the notebook that she had put together to organize her notes, research, records of her doctor appointments and the many healthcare tasks that we all need to do, I told her that I wished that I had been so organized when I was dealing with my breast cancer years before and how helpful that would have been. I suggested that it would be very useful to others if she could show us how to do it. First she gave us After Shock: From Cancer Diagnosis to Healing. Now she's completed and revised the organizer I had in mind—and how fine it is!

My wish is that My Hope & Focus Cancer Organizer eases your process and lightens your load as you meet the various challenges following your initial diagnosis, a recurrence or termination of treatment.

Blessings,
Puja Thomson

Thank you for purchasing
My Hope & Focus Cancer Organizer

Second Revised Edition 2022
ISBN 978-1-928663-15-7 $19.95

My Hope & Focus Cancer Organizer is also available from Roots & Wings as an
E-book in downloadable PDF format. $7.95

Other titles from ROOTS & WINGS:

Track Your Truth—Discover Your Authentic Self
Paperback ISBN 978-1-928663-10-2 $17.95   E-book ISBN 978-1-928663-16-4 $4.95

After Shock: From Cancer Diagnosis to Healing (Second revised edition 2021)
Paperback ISBN 978-1-928663-17-1 $19.95

Roots & Wings for Strength and Freedom
Guided imagery and meditations to transform your life

• CD   ISBN 978-1-928663-08-9 $15.00
MP3 (check online at rootsnwings.com/store)
• Paperback workbook Revised Edition   ISBN 978-1-928663-06-5 $19.95
• Workbook & CD Revised Edition   ISBN 978-1-928663-07-2 $24.00

My Health & Wellness Organizer
(Revised edition 2022) ISBN 978-1-928663-14-0 *$19.95*
Also available as an e-book in downloadable PDF format from Roots & Wings $7.95

TO ORDER
Any of the above titles or for general inquiries:

845-255-2278
www.rootsnwings.com
Also available from local bookstores and online retailers.

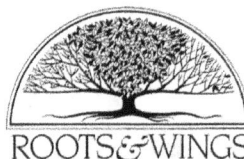

ROOTS&WINGS

ROOTS & WINGS PUBLISHING
P. O. Box 1081, New Paltz, NY 12561   info@rootsnwings.com